Anoint Yourself With Oil

For Radiant Health

David Richard

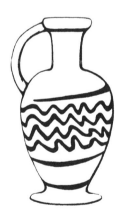

Vital Health Publishing

P.O. Box 544
Bloomingdale, IL 60108
(630) 876-0426

Cover Layout and Typography by Studio 2D,
Champaign, IL.

Printing and Production by United Graphics,
Mattoon, IL.

ISBN 1-890612-01-04

Cover Illustration: Etruscan Pitcher
used for perfumed oil (C. 500-600 BC)

Cover and interior illustrations
by John Scott Murdoch.

With gratitude to the ancient ones
who understood the value of hygiene
toward health and well-being.

*"If you forget me, think of our gifts
to Aphrodite and all the loveliness
that we shared . . . myrrh poured on
your head and on the soft mats girls
with all that they most wished for
beside them"*

—Sappho

Contents

Anoint Yourself With Oil For Radiant Health

CHAPTER 1

Introduction

*Hygeia: in Greek Mythology, the
goddess of health, daughter of
Aesculapius [God of Medicine].*

—Websters Unabridged Dictionary

*"Nature is the True Physician,
Hygiene is Her Handmaid."*

—Susanna Way Dodds, M.D. (1915)

Every year, millions of dollars in advertising are spent to convince you to moisturize and nourish your skin with a variety of cosmetic cremes, moisturizers and gels or to dry the naturally-occurring oils in your skin with a variety of powders, soaps and sprays. Nearly all of these products are overpriced, ineffective and laden with synthetically-derived chemicals. Even the majority of so-called 'natural' alternatives have a variety of synthetic additives or natural substances which have been chemically-modified to create a more 'appealing' finished product. In addition, much of the advertising tries to convince you that oils, including your own body's sebaceous oils, are harmful because they block your pores or contribute to a 'greasy' appearance. Nothing, of course, could be further from the truth.

The truth is that your skin and much of the rest of your body has two primary needs in addition to protein to remain in good health: water and oil. Without these two substances, the skin becomes withered and dried, and the underlying metabolism is similarly affected.

Oil Therapy, hereafter called Hygienic Oil Therapy, is an ancient hygienic and therapeutic practice which has been used by cultures around the world for millennia in the pursuit of health and beauty. Modern science confirms that the nutrients present in unrefined oils are absorbed into and through skin and provide nourishment to a variety of organ and glandular systems. Foremost among these nutrients are the essential fatty acids (EFAs) which are considered essential because they cannot be manufactured in the human body. High quality vegetable oils, such as olive, flax, hemp, sesame and almond contain one or both of the EPAs in the Omega-6 or Omega-3 families. They also include the natural antioxidants, Vitamins A and E, and a number of other important nutrients.

The health benefits of Hygienic Oil Therapy, also known as anointment in its historical and religious contexts, are significant and varied. It provides primary nourishment for the skin and helps to heal and cleanse it. It also helps to soothe and relax the nerves, nourish the heart and brain, and lubricate the joints in addition to providing nutrients essential to the creation and functioning of hormones within the endocrine system. EFAs have also been shown to reduce blood pressure, lower cholesterol and triglyceride levels and reduce the growth rate of tumors in breast cancer.

This book describes one method of ingesting EFAs and other important nutrients into the body at the same time the skin is being nourished and cleansed. I have called this method Hygienic Oil Therapy since I know of no more descriptive name which is faithful to all of the traditions from which it is derived. Its essence is simple: A daily self-massage is used to cover the body with a thin film of nutritive oil which is gradually absorbed into the skin. Hygienic Oil Therapy is relaxing, self-nourishing and healthful. And it costs less than thirty-five cents a day to accrue its benefits.

The rest of this book will describe the traditions from which Hygienic Oil Therapy is derived, the science of subcutaneous or transdermal absorption, essential fatty acid metabolism and other nutritive properties of oils, types and grades of oil from which you can choose, the daily practice of Hygienic Oil Therapy through self-massage, adding herbs and Aromatherapy to your routine according to your own instinct or the Aryuvedic tradition of doshas (body types), and how this practice can help you to fast more effectively and with less stress. There is also a question-and-answer section to help you with common concerns in getting started. My hope is that you will add this healthy habit to your daily routine and it will benefit you as much as it has benefited me.

> *"The only useful part of medicine is hygiene. And the hygiene is itself less a science than a virtue."*

> —Rousseau

CHAPTER 2

The Tradition

*'Anoint' : from the Latin inungere,
to smear on. Replaced the Old
English, smerian. See also unguent,
ointment.*

—Webster's Unabridged Dictionary

*"There the Graces washed her and
anointed her with immortal olive oil,
such as is poured on the ever-living
gods, and put her in charming
clothes, a wonder to behold."*

—Homer, *The Odyssey*,
Book VIII, 364-366

The tradition of anointment with oil in religious consecration and worship is both ancient and widespread. Anointment has also been widely
practiced as a means of healing the sick and as an embalming technique in burying the dead. According to S.G.F. Brandon in *Man, Myth
and Magic,* the religious usage of anointing oils and unguents had its
origin in the daily hygienic practices of people who, in ritual circum-
stances, accorded special meaning to different oils, salves and ointments.
He comments on those traditions as follows:

"The Egyptians, for example, made much use of perfumed ointments
as pleasing emollients: the celebrated golden throne found in the tomb
of Tutankhamen depicts, on its back panel, the queen anointing the
young King; on festal occasions the Egyptians wore cones of perfumed
ointment on their heads, which gradually melted in the heat and
anointed their bodies. Consequently, in the daily toilet-ritual performed in temples for the pleasure of their gods, their cult images, as
representatives of themselves, were solemnly anointed. Similar toilet

ceremonies are performed in the Hindu temple. . . . Greek mythology also reveals that the gods were thought to delight in fragrant unguents as mortals did. The goddess Hera, seeking to win the favor of Zeus, carefully prepared herself by bathing in ambrosia and anointing herself with perfumed oil (Iliad, book 14)."

Historical evidence reveals that both the Greeks and Romans utilized oil and perfumed oil in their celebrated baths as did the Aztec civilization in the new world. Eskimos, restricted to animal resources, rubbed the oil of seals onto their skin to keep it smooth and supple and to help fortify themselves against the elements.

Within the Judeo-Christian tradition, anointment with oil conveys a religious significance similar to that of other cultures and reflects, undoubtedly, the daily health habits of the Jewish people. The first Old Testament reference to anointment occurs in the Law of Moses and describes the consecration of the high priest. Similar instructions are given for the anointment of the articles of worship within the tabernacle, for the anointment of the king, and for the anointment of sanctified articles within the temple at Jerusalem. The oil used, on the majority of these occasions, was a holy oil whose contents are described in Exodus 30. It is described as being a high quality olive oil, sweetened and perfumed with spices of liquid myrrh (a tree resin), sweet-smelling cinnamon, sweet-smelling cane and cassia (perhaps a gum).

There are nearly three hundred biblical references to various forms of anointment with oil. The Psalms refer to the "oil of gladness" and "oil to make the face shine." The Proverbs recommend "ointment and perfume to delight the heart." And the prophet Isaiah refers to the "oil of joy." Most people know the story of the prostitute, Mary Magdelene, who anointed Jesus' head with fragrant oil and wiped his feet with her hair. Jesus has been historically called the Lord's Anointed. In this connection, the title Christ comes from the Latin Christos, meaning 'The Anointed'. It is relevant to note that Jesus' disciples healed the sick as they anointed them with oil.

Within the Catholic tradition of Christianity, anointment remains a vital aspect of the rituals of worship and healing. According to the treatises of Cyril of Jerusalem and Hippolytus (fourth and fifth century), candidates for baptism should be completely anointed with exorcised oil prior to immersion. Hippolytus adds a second anointing with sanc-

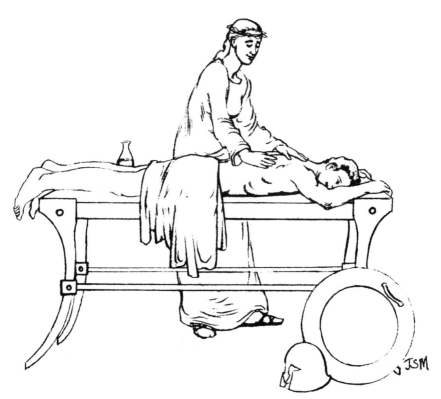

Polykaste Anoints Telemachos, *The Odyssey,* Book III, 464-468.

tified oil following the immersion. This tradition was later reduced to a partial anointment and extended into the rite of confirmation also. The ritual of the anointing of the sick or the dying (unction of the Sick and Extreme Unction) is also a part of the Catholic Tradition. The authority for the rite is given in James, Chapter 5: "Is any man sick? Let him call for the elders of the church, and let them pray over him, anointing him with oil in the name of the Lord. And the prayer of faith will save the sick, and the Lord will raise him up. And if he has committed sins, he will be forgiven."

The Judeao-Christian tradition of the anointment of royalty was historically extended and represented in the ceremonial anointment of both the French and English Kings. According to legend, the French tradition began with the baptism of Clovis (c 465-511) who reportedly founded the French monarchy. It was believed that a vial of consecrated oil descended from heaven for the anointing of the King. According to Brandon, "Every French King, down to the ill-fated Louis XVI, was anointed at his coronation with Chrism that contained a tiny fragment of the solidified oil of Clovis." Not to be outdone by their French rivals, a vial of anointing oil was "miraculously" found in the tower of London during the reign of Richard II. It was identified as the oil given by the Virgin Mary to St. Thomas of Canterbury for the purpose of anointing the kings of England. Before Richard could make use of this divine gift, he was deposed and it was used in the coronation of his supplanter, Henry IV. While the French tradition of anointment with oil was lost with the monarchy in their revolution, the English tradition remains a vital part of their coronation ceremony.

In India, anointment with oil is both a relic of the Hindu religion and a living practice of one of the most ancient systems of organized medicine, Aryuveda. A daily self-massage (Abhyanga) using a prepared oil according to body type, or Dosha, is an important aspect of maintaining health and balance according to Aryuvedic tradition. It is particularly important in the cold, dry season of late fall to early spring, known as the Vata season. Vata also represents one of the three basic body types which is generally characterized as being thin, quick, dry, cold and rough. The Pitta Dosha is characterized as being hot, sharp, moist and sour-smelling. And the Kapha Dosha is characterized as being heavy, sweet, steady, soft and slow. While people are considered to be a mixture of all of these characteristics, one or two doshas usually predominate and are used by Aryuvedic practitioners for diagnostic and prescriptive purposes.

In regard to the daily oil massage, this differentiation results in the use of different herbal combinations, infused into the oil, to balance the Doshas. These will be discussed in greater detail in Chapter 6 where the practice of Hygienic Oil Therapy is described in relationship to Aromatherapy. For now, it is enough to know that sesame oil, purified and "cured" at approximately 220°F, is the oil of choice for most conditions in Aryuvedic medicine. Used daily, the Abhyanga is thought to help balance all three body types, to help relax the nerves and to contribute toward the production of endocrine hormones. According to Deepak Chopra, MD, the practice is traditionally recognized as having many benefits: "In Ancient times, Chavaka lavished praise on the practice of Abhyanga, holding that it rejuvenates the skin, tones the muscles, eliminates impurities, and promotes youthfulness."

Another Aryuvedic practice using oil is the Shirodhana in which "warm, herbalized sesame oil is slowly dripped onto the forehead to profoundly relax the nervous system and balance the (energies) of the brain."

Whether used in religious ritual or secular hygienic practice, it is traditionally-recognized that oil has healing as well as cleansing properties. The regard that led personal anointment to be elevated to the anointment of kings and priests gives all the more credence to the original hygienic practice which, I believe, is common to all indigenous people, from the South Sea Islanders to the Eskimos of Gnome.

> *"Not all the water in the rough, rude sea can wash balm from an anointed King."*
>
> —Shakespeare, Richard II,
> Act III, ii, 54

Anoint Yourself With Oil For Radiant Health

CHAPTER 3

The Science

*"Essential substances, including
healing fats, must be obtained in
optimal quantities to maintain
optimal health"*

—Udo Erasmus

Hygienic Oil Therapy is a practice which modern science has not fully caught up with, probably because there is little financial incentive to investigate it. Nevertheless, scientists have defined three areas of investigation which, taken as unit, provide a reasonable understanding of how Hygienic Oil Therapy works. These areas are: the Physiology of the Skin, the Principle of Transdermal Absorption and the Nutritional Properties of Unrefined Oils.

The Science of the Skin

The largest single organ of the body is not the heart, the brain or the lungs — it is the skin. The skin serves as a primary barrier of protection between our internal organs and the outside world. It is the point of physical contact (or sense) between those inner and outer worlds. It is also one of our most important organs of elimination. In addition, the skin works with other organs of the body to help regulate both our temperature and our fluid balance through the process of perspiration.

As a protective barrier, our skin depends upon a thin film of oil. This film is common to both plants and animals. Plants store oil in the protective coating of their seeds. Animals maintain a coating of oil on their skins. In both cases, the function of the oil is to keep toxins and harmful bacteria outside and to keep valuable nutrients and fluids within. Since the fatty acids in sebaceous oil have a mildly negative pH value, they also help to support the acid mantle of the skin which is a primary deterrent to potentially harmful bacteria, viruses, fungi and other microbes.

As a sense organ, the skin is rich in nerve endings which respond to variations in pressure and temperature with a wonderful variety of sensations, both mild and intense. Much of the pain we experience, as well as the pleasure, comes from the nerves of the skin. Without this pain, we would subject our bodies to untold amounts of trauma, as has been demonstrated by those who have lost their tactile sense. Physiologically, the nerve endings, located in the papillae of the skin, depend upon a wide variety of nutrients to keep them functioning optimally. Among these nutrients are the EFAs, vitamins, minerals and phytonutrients present in unrefined nutritive oils.

As an organ of elimination, the skin depends upon the sweat glands and the oil (sebaceous) glands. The sweat glands are associated with skin pores and are concentrated in the less hairy areas of the body. The oil glands are associated with the hair follicles and are concentrated in the more hairy areas of the body. The sweat glands secrete mostly water and mineral salts, together with waste products of cellular respiration. The oil glands secrete an oily, semi-fluid substance called sebum whose primary function is to lubricate and cleanse the skin and hair. In addition, some of the fat-bound toxins in the system are eliminated through the sebum. This, as much as any external influence, may well account for many "diseases of the skin" since the health of the skin is predicated upon the health of the individual as a whole.

In terms of the the skin's regulatory function, toward maintaining a healthy temperature and fluid balance within the body, perspiration is more important than oil secretion. However, Hygienic Oil Therapy can help to warm the body by introducing-beneficial fats which burn more slowly than carbohydrates. On a per weight basis, nutritional oil (healthy fat) supplies nearly twice the amount of energy (calories) as is supplied by carbohydrates. And unlike the harmful saturated or hydrogenated fats, these oils contribute to our health rather than to degenerative conditions and diseases of our systems. The warming effect of oils and fats is part of the reason for the Eskimo people rubbing animal fats on their skin. The comparative health of these people also illustrates that different kinds of fats and oils have benefits within different climatic conditions.

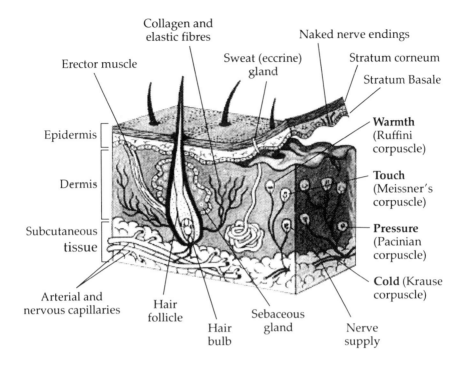

Collagen and elastic fibres
Naked nerve endings
Erector muscle
Sweat (eccrine) gland
Stratum corneum
Stratum Basale
Epidermis
Dermis
Subcutaneous tissue
Warmth (Ruffini corpuscle)
Touch (Meissner's corpuscle)
Pressure (Pacinian corpuscle)
Cold (Krause corpuscle)
Arterial and nervous capillaries
Hair follicle
Hair bulb
Sebaceous gland
Nerve supply

Transdermal Absorption

Science has traditionally held the view that the skin is a barrier rather than an organ of metabolism. It has further held than any absorption through the skin is based on diffusion and is fixed at a constant rate. Recent evidence has shown that neither of these assumptions is true. In the first place, the skin is alive and is capable of making distinctions of what to absorb and what to eliminate. It is also capable of making biological transformations or "extensive" metabolism according to Jerry Hall, one of the co-authors of a study exploring transdermal absorption which was conducted at Oak Ridge (Tenn.) National Laboratory. This study showed that the rate of absorption of a hormone (testosterone) was 12 to 16 times greater than that of a toxic chemical (benzo [a] pyrene) It further showed that the rate of absorption of the toxin was greater in hairy mice than skinless mice. The researchers concluded that this was because the hairy mice had more sebaceous glands where metabolism of the fat-seeking toxin occurred. In simple terms, the skin drinks in what it needs and tries to resist foreign or toxic matter. It is a selective barrier with metabolic factories in the sebaceous glands.

These holes in the barrier, together with the constant diffusion of substances through the skin are the basis of transdermal patches, one of the newest delivery systems for medication. According to the Medical Encyclopedia of Rush-Presbyterian–St. Luke's Medical Center, trandermal infusion of medication

"is a technique for applying medication in which a gel-like strip of material is placed on the skin. The medication is then absorbed through the skin at a constant rate. This technique is often used in the administration of estrogen, nitroglycerin, and scopolamine . . . as well as nicotine for smoking cessation."

Many more patches are on their way to market, including those containing cardiovascular, arthritic and anti-inflammatory drugs.

In terms of Hygienic Oil Therapy, transdermal medicine is further evidence that the skin is capable of drinking in nutrients as well as absorbing toxins or drugs. As Thomas J. Franz, MD and director of clinical investigation at Hoffman La Roche says, "The skin is like a sponge. It's safest to assume that everything gets through to a degree." And, thankfully, this includes the nutritional oils and their EFAs.

The Nutrition of Unrefined Oils

Unrefined nutritional oils can be defined as those which are intended for human consumption and have not had their nutrients processed out of them through the application of heat or chemicals. I will describe how to select a high-quality nutritional oil and some of the processing techniques and their related terminology in the following chapter. For now, let us turn our attention to the essential fatty acids (EFAs) and their role in human nutrition.

Seeds and nuts are the primary plant sources of nutritive oil and EFAs. As indicated previously, their oil provides a protective barrier for preserving the nutrients and moisture within the seed. However, it does much more than this. The oil also provides nourishment for the early growth of the seed in the same way that an infant is nourished by a mother's milk. This vegetable 'formula' is responsible for the growth of the seed until it can begin to extract nutrients from the soil and convert them to usable form through the energy of the sun. Among the ingredients in this formula are the two essential fatty acids, alpha-linolenic acid (LNA) and linoleic acid (LA). A third fatty acid, gamma-linolenic acid (GLA) may be considered essential, in practical terms, because many individuals lack the necessary nutrients to convert LA to GLA.

LNA and LA are known as "essential fatty acids" because the body must have them and because they cannot be manufactured from other fatty acids in the body. They fall into two categories: the Omega-3 fatty acids, represented by LNA, and the Omega-6 fatty acids, represented by LA. The Omega-3 fatty acids are more generally associated with fish oils which makes finding a rich source of LNA particularly important to a vegetarian diet. The Omega-6 fatty acids also include GLA whose association with LA I have previously noted.

Many individuals are deficient in one or both of the essential fatty acids. This deficiency is undoubtedly due to the high levels of consumption of refined oils which have little of the EFAs remaining in them, of saturated fats in the form of meat and dairy products, and of altered or hydrogenated fats as are commonly used in margarines and snack products. This replacement has occurred to the detriment of our health and well being and has a very high degree of correlation with the degenerative diseases which afflict us: heart disease, arthritis, immune disorders and cancer. In addition, deficiencies are widespread in the nutrient cofactors necessary for the conversion of EFAs (see chart on following page).

Women, in particular, are vulnerable to EFA deficiency, as well as GLA deficiency, since more of their body weight is typically stored as fat than that of men. Moreover, their entire menstrual cycle is regulated by a hormone, estrogen, which is derived from essential fatty acids. This may be the basis for research which shows that EFA ingestion reduces the rate of growth of tumors in cases of breast cancer.

Essential fatty acids nourish a number of vital systems and functions with the body. Their primary functions are: assisting the production of energy through the process of oxidation, helping to transport oxygen across cell walls and membranes in order to fuel this process, helping to produce hemoglobin for healthy red blood cells, assisting the development of permeable membranes within and around each cell, pro-

EFA Conversion to Prostaglandins

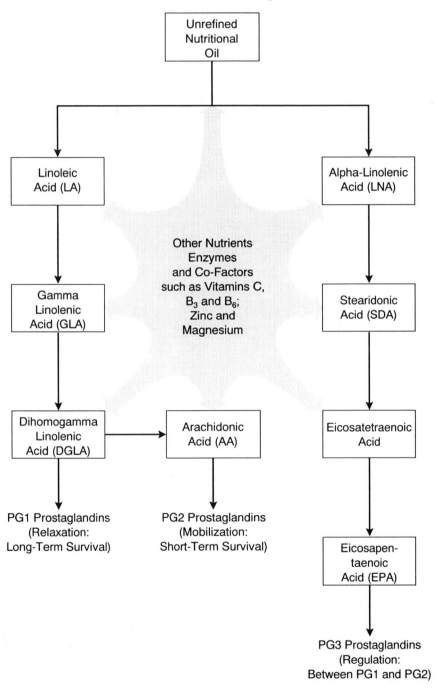

Unrefined Nutritional Oil

Linoleic Acid (LA)

Alpha-Linolenic Acid (LNA)

Other Nutrients Enzymes and Co-Factors such as Vitamins C, B₃ and B₆; Zinc and Magnesium

Gamma Linolenic Acid (GLA)

Stearidonic Acid (SDA)

Dihomogamma Linolenic Acid (DGLA)

Arachidonic Acid (AA)

Eicosatetraenoic Acid

PG1 Prostaglandins (Relaxation: Long-Term Survival)

PG2 Prostaglandins (Mobilization: Short-Term Survival)

Eicosapentaenoic Acid (EPA)

PG3 Prostaglandins (Regulation: Between PG1 and PG2)

Anoint Yourself With Oil For Radiant Health

moting recovery from fatigue, helping to synthesize the hormone-like prostaglandins, promoting growth and normal development, assisting cell division, and a host of other activities too numerous to list.

The role of EFAs in creating prostaglandins is a particularly exciting subject in relationship to nutritional oil therapy. Prostaglandins are the short-lived regulating substances which govern many of our body's functions. They are composed almost entirely of the EFAs which we consume in the form of nutritional oil. Among their many hormone-like functions, one group of prostaglandins has been shown to reduce the adhesiveness of blood platelets, reduce sodium and excess fluid from the kidneys, improve circulation and lower blood pressure, slow cholesterol production, decrease inflammation, improve nerve functioning, increase insulin efficiency, and strengthen the immune system. Another group is responsible for the survival response in which many of these activities are beneficially reversed. As a whole, prostaglandins help to maintain the subtle balance of internal and external forces we call 'health'.

We have already considered the role of the sebaceous glands in providing sebum to lubricate, nourish and cleanse the skin and hair. When the healthy EFAs in our bodies are deficient, the skin becomes dry and the hair becomes listless. This is why the EFAs are often recommended for skin and hair problems and are included in related dietary supplements. It is possible, however, to deal with these problems more directly by massaging a nutritional oil into the skin. The skin is moisturized and softened (one of the meanings of emollient), the sebaceous glands are refreshed and given a rest, and the EFAs and other nutrients are absorbed into the system. Udo Erasmus tells us in his informative book, Fats that Heal, Fats that Kill:

> "Beautiful skin requires EFAs. Skin properly nourished with EFAs is smoother, feels softer, shows less of the above conditions [listed as acne, skin rash, black heads and whiteheads, bumpy skin, eczema, dry skin and 'greasy' skin], is infected less easily, and looks radiant. It also ages more slowly and remains wrinkle-free longer."

There is an abundance of evidence to support the role of EFAs in the maintenance of a healthy heart and cardiovascular system and in the treatment of related disorders. EFAs have successfully helped treat coronary heart disease, reduce blood pressure, help reverse arteriosclerosis, and lower cholesterol and triglyceride levels. Erasmus tells us: "Highly unsaturated, natural fatty acids (EFAs) keep saturated fatty acids dispersed by preventing them from aggregating. They are also necessary for transporting cholesterol. In this function, EFAs are first hooked up (esterified) with the cholesterol."

In addition, EFAs occur at high levels in brain tissues and nerve cells and have been shown to assist in many vital brain and nerve functions. Among these functions are the development of the brain in infants and children, the ability to learn and recall information, the transmission of nerve impulses in the central nervous system, and the ability to accurately perform cognitive and motor tasks. In particular, research performed by Dr. William Connor, Professor of Medicine at Oregon Health Sciences University, has shown that EFAs are essential for the normal function and development of the brain.

Finally, EFAs have been shown to have a soothing, lubricating effect in the prevention of arthritis and in the treatment of inflammatory conditions of the digestive tract and skin such as eczema or psoriasis. Erasmus states: "Essential Fatty Acids (EFAs) are necessary to produce secretions that lubricate our joints. They are also required to build and deposit bone material, and used to transport minerals."

In addition to EFAs, unrefined nutritional oils also contain measurable quantities of the fat-soluble antioxidants Beta Carotene and Vitamin E as well as trace amounts of various minerals and phytonutrients. The antioxidants are used by the seed or nut to prevent the oil from rancidifying, and the other nutrients are trace elements which have been retained in the pressing. While none of these nutrients is present in large amounts, they are synergistically balanced and combined in a way which maximizes the health and vitality of the next generation of plant life from which they came. And so, they contribute to our health and vitality.

> "Let it enter his body . . . like oil into
> his bones"
>
> —Ps. 109:18

Anoint Yourself With Oil For Radiant Health

Types and Grades of Oil

*"Oleum (oil) comes from the Greek
word Elaion both words meaning
"olive oil" or "another oily substance." Elaion, in turn, derives from
Elaia, "olive tree, olive."*

—From Word Mysteries and Histories

Processing Of Oils

Certain seeds, nuts and plants are processed in a variety of ways to yield nutritional oil. Historically, pressing was the method that was used to extract oil from the fibrous portion of the seed or plant. In the case of olives, a number of pressings are used to successively remove a larger percentage of the oil. The first pressing yields the finest oil and the term "extra virgin" is applied. In addition to olive oil, a number of other oils are obtained by pressing. While this method is less efficient and therefore more costly than other methods of extraction, it retains the highest percentage of nutrients in the finished oil.

Cold or temperature-controlled pressing refers to the temperature at which the oil is pressed. Since many tons of pressure are often used in pressing the seeds or nuts, heat is generated which may destroy some or all of the delicate nutrients in the oil. Oils which are pressed at low temperature in the absence of oxygen and light are of the highest quality. They are usually darker in color than other oils and require refrigeration from the moment they are pressed. Look for these oils in the refrigerated section of your health food store. Olive Oil, with its higher percentage of monounsaturated fats, is often pressed at low-temperature yet remains shelf stable. Do not rely, however, on the labeling claim "cold-pressed" since it has no technical definition.

Solvent extraction uses a chemical solvent to "attack" the seed and separate the oil. This method is used because it is inexpensive and yields more oil. The solvents may vary in their toxicity from simple alcohol to hexane or heptane. Nearly all of the solvent evaporates or is separated from the finished oil. However, a small portion of the solvent remains. And, as we have seen, whatever is placed on the skin enters the body. In addition, many of the delicate nutrients of the seed or plant may be destroyed by exposure to these chemicals. Therefore, solvent-extracted oils are not recommended for external use any more than for internal use.

The refining of vegetable oils continues well beyond the process of solvent extraction. Since natural antioxidants are removed or destroyed by the application of solvents, synthetic stabilizers are added to preserve the oil from rancidity. A degumming step removes the phospholipids, including the lecithin. Refining, bleaching and deodorizing steps apply chemicals and heat to the oil, further removing valuable nutrients. The end result of the refining process is an oil which is as devoid of nutritive value as white bread or refined sugar. The process also results in harmful substances called trans-fatty acids being formed in the oil which have been implicated in many degenerative conditions of the body. In addition, there is evidence that the refining process and resulting depletion of nutrients may be responsible for some of the conflicting results and conclusions regarding the health benefits of food-grade oils.

Virtually every oil you find in the supermarket and even some of the oils in health food stores are solvent-extracted. These oils have the advantage of being shelf-stable and non-rancidifying for a much longer period of time than a nutrient-rich unrefined oil. Only if the term 'unrefined' is used on the label or the label clearly states that the oil was not solvent-extracted can you be certain of its nutritive value. This may include a category of 'pressed' oils which are shelf-stable. While not as beneficial as the virgin olive oil or refrigerated nutritional oils, these have the advantage of a lower price together with some nutritional benefit.

Cosmetic, Food and Organic Grades

Cosmetic oils are produced to meet a different set of standards than food-grade oils. Generally, they are solvent-extracted. Unless the label tells you otherwise, assume that the oil has been solvent-extracted and look for a superior grade of oil.

Food-grade oils are processed for human consumption. Since we have already seen that the skin 'consumes' what is put upon it, food-grade oils are more appropriate than cosmetic oils. However, the issue of refined versus unrefined oil applies, as has been previously discussed.

Organic oil refers to the growing conditions of the seed or plant. If the plant has been grown in soil which has not been treated by chemical pesticides, germicides or fertilizers, it may be called an organic oil. Usually, an independent association certifies organic products. Look for their seal on the label as a mark of authenticity. Otherwise, the term 'organic' is only a labeling claim of the manufacturer. Some of the more common designations are OCIA (Organic Crop Improvement Association), OGBA (Organic Growers and Buyers Association) and CCOF (California Certified Organic Farmers). In addition, both California and Texas have comprehensive organic regulatory codes which are enforced by state authorities.

Organic, unrefined oil is the highest quality oil you can buy. It represents the richest nutrient profile and the strictest standards for pesticide and herbicide levels due to the organic farming and certification methods. And it represents the most gentle and healthy processing of the seeds or nuts in order to preserve the nutrients and to avoid the addition of toxic chemicals or the creation of harmful trans-fatty acids.

Varieties of Oils

Every oil has its own special properties. I will list some of the major oils and outline but a few of their properties.

General Purpose Oils

These oils are the most useful for Hygienic Oil Therapy and are priced so that they can be used over the entire body.

OLIVE OIL • The healthiest olive oil is labeled 'virgin' or 'extra virgin'. This means that the oil is unrefined and has been mechanically pressed without the destructive effects of heat or chemical additives. 'Extra Virgin' refers to an unrefined oil which is from the first pressing of the olives and is the most nutritionally rich.

Olive oil has the oldest tradition of usage of any of the oils and is most closely associated with the development of civilization.

Olive Oil is rich in monounsaturated fatty acids (80%) and is subsequently more stable than other oils containing more of the EFAs. Because the oil comes from the soft fruit of olives, it is the only mass-marketed unrefined oil. In other words, it is the only healthy oil, in my opinion, that you can buy at the supermarket.

While relatively deficient in EFAs, Virgin Olive Oil has a host of nutrients which account for its benefits in preventing cardiovascular disease, in improving brain and neurological functioning, and in reducing the mutagenicity of cells and improving their structural integrity. In addition, it is an excellent emollient for the skin. Some of the nutrients in olive oil, according to Erasmus, are:

> "the antioxidants, beta-carotene and Vitamin E; chlorophyll, squalene and various phytosterols; and triterpenic modified sterols, polyphenols and over 100 other volatile organic compounds. Refined olive oil contains relatively few of these nutrients due to over-processing."

One additional phytonutrient, oleuropin, is present in unrefined olive oil which has anecdotally shown benefit in treating HIV-positive patients as well as anti-microbial activity and therapeutic value in cases of dermatitis and psoriasis. Since it is more concentrated in the leaves, an olive leaf extract may have greater efficacy than the extra virgin oil.

SESAME OIL • Sesame oil is the oil of choice within the Aryuvedic tradition of Abhyanga. Sesame oil is a thick oil with a heavy odor. Like olive oil, it is rich in monounsaturates, and it is also a significant source of linoleic acid (LA). It is more warming than olive oil, especially when it comes from roasted seeds or if it is cured by the Aryuvedic method. 'Curing' consists of briefly heating the oil to approximately the temperature of boiling water for a few seconds. You can avoid starting a fire (oil burns) by placing a quarter cup of oil in a container of water that has just been boiled. Sesame oil is considered both balancing and relaxing, according to Deepak Chopra. Note that roasting the sesame

Anoint Yourself With Oil For Radiant Health

seeds sacrifices some of the heat-sensitive nutrients of the oil. Consequently, a non-roasted sesame oil is preferable.

ALMOND OIL • Sweet Almond Oil has been traditionally used by massage therapists to lubricate the skin during a therapeutic massage. Because of its high oleic acid content, almond oil is a monounsaturated oil which is relatively stable. It is also rich in Vitamin E. Almond oil is a light oil with healing properties for dry, itching or inflammatory skin conditions such as eczema.

FLAX OIL • The use of flax seeds as a source of nutrition is ancient, undoubtedly pre-dating the earliest historical records of its cultivation by the Babylonians around 5000 BC. The Egyptians, Greeks, Romans, Indian (Hindi) and early European cultures were also known to have prized flax, perhaps as much for its fibrous stalks in making linen as for the nutritive value of its seeds.

Flax seeds yield a robust oil with excellent nutritive properties. There are many fine organic, cold-pressed flax oil products on the market which are rich and golden in color and have the warming qualities of flax seeds. This warming quality is common to many oils derived from seeds which grow in cold climates. Flax oil contains an excellent balance of fatty acids, including significant amounts of alpha-linolenic acid (LNA). It is also rich in Vitamins A and E and retains a small portion of plant lignans through its pressing, which are important because of their anti-microbial and anti-cancerous properties. In addition, it contains trace amounts of Vitamins C, B_1, and B_2 and all of the major and trace minerals.

Using flax oil is a treat because of its nutty, buttery aroma. Look for it in the refrigerated section of your health food store and be certain to keep it refrigerated at home. This will keep it fresh and healthful.

HEMP OIL • Udo Erasmus lists hemp oil, from the marijuana plant, as the most balanced and nutritious of all the seed oils. It is rich in the EFAs: alpha-linolenic acid (LNA), and linoleic acid (LA) as well as providing a measure of gamma-linolenic acid (GLA). According to Erasmus, its unusually well-balanced EFA profile means that one could use it for a lifetime without ever suffering from an EFA deficiency. With its light green color and a taste and smell reminiscent of sunflower oil, hemp oil is an excellent choice for Hygienic Oil Therapy. Do not worry about hallucinatory side-effects because it contains no THC and is perfectly legal.

SUNFLOWER OIL • The oil of sunflower seeds is light and rich in nutrients. Sixty-five percent of its fat content is in the Omega-6 fatty acids, and it contains measurable quantities of Zinc and Vitamin E. Like many highly unsaturated oils, sunflower oil should be packaged in an opaque container rather than a transparent bottle in order to protect the light-sensitive EFAs and antioxidants. Organic, unrefined sunflower oil is a healthy treat which benefits dry and delicate skin types. There are hi-oleic varieties of sunflower oil which I would not recommend for Hygienic Oil Therapy. Hi-oleic oils are more stable than traditional varieties for cooking purposes but are less nutritionally rich.

SOYBEAN OIL • Unrefined soy oil is nutrient-rich, light and mildly scented. Unfortunately it is also rare since the oil content of soybeans is low (18%) compared to other sources, and pressing yields less oil than solvent extraction. If you can find a high-quality oil, give it a try since it contains measurable quantities of lecithin, phytosterols, isoflavones, genestein and other phytonutrients in addition to a rich balance of fatty acids. Soy oil is particularly rich in the Omega-6 Fatty Acids (50%).

CANOLA OIL • Derived from a special low-erucic acid breed of rape seeds, canola oil (an abbreviation of Canadian oil, where it was developed) is primarily a monounsaturated oil which has less EFAs than some of the polyunsaturated oils. Nevertheless, it is an important nutritional oil which is appropriate for use in Hygienic Oil Therapy in its unrefined form. The high-oleic varieties of canola oil are more stable yet have still less of the EFAs. A light, mildly-scented oil, canola oil penetrates the skin quickly and offers a healthy amount of linoleic acid (LA).

PUMPKIN SEED OIL • Unrefined pumpkin seed oil is green in color, due to its chlorophyll content, and rich in important nutrients. Its high content of linoleic acid (45-60%), magnesium and zinc have made it an important ingredient in encapsulated formulations for prostate problems and for men in general. Note that zinc is one of the nutrients necessary to convert LA to GLA, and GLA is necessary in the synthesis of the hormone-like prostaglandins. In Hygienic Oil Therapy, pumpkin seed oil is an excellent choice for both men and women when it can be obtained unrefined and fresh. If it tastes or smells 'bitter,' it has become rancid and is no longer suitable for use.

SAFFLOWER OIL • As with most of the seed oils, unrefined safflower oil is rich in linoleic acid. However, compared to flax oil, it lacks alpha-linolenic acid. Because it rancidifies quickly, safflower oil is perhaps better used internally than externally. The hi-oleic variety of safflower oil is more stable but better suited for cooking than for Hygienic Oil Therapy.

Specialty Oils

These oils have nutritive properties which may be most applicable to people with special needs or problems. They may also be too expensive for general usage. It is possible, however, to blend these oils into the General Purpose Oils for their added benefits.

EVENING PRIMROSE OIL • EPO has a high content of Gamma-Linolenic Acid (GLA) which is generally deficient in our population and is especially important for women. Note that excellent results have been obtained using evening primrose oil to minimize premenstrual (PMS) symptoms as well as other problems associated with female hormonal imbalances. GLA helps to promote healthy skin and to repair inflamed, dry or damaged skin. Its cost may make it most appropriate for facial oil treatments where it discourages dry skin and premature aging. However, it may also be helpful in conditions of psoriasis and dermatitis. Use only a cold-pressed EPO to avoid solvent residues.

BORAGE OIL • Like evening primrose oil, borage oil has an unusually high content of Gamma-Linolenic Acid (GLA) which the body readily converts to prostaglandins. As a result, borage oil stimulates skin cell activity and encourages cell regeneration. Borage oil can be added to other nutritional oils to increase their benefit, or it can be used directly to rejuvenate the skin.

ROSE HIP SEED OIL • Rose hip seed oil is notable for its relatively high content of Vitamin C and citrus bioflavanoids in addition to a healthy spectrum of EFAs. As a result, it is recommended for strengthening the collagen of the skin in order to reduce scarring, to heal burns and to promote regeneration of skin cells. A more costly emollient, rose hip seed oil is excellent for limited application — onto the face, onto delicate, dry and exposed areas, and onto areas of damage such as scar tissue or broken capillaries.

JOJOBA OIL • Jojoba oil has gained its reputation by helping to restore hair growth in cases of premature baldness. It is very similar in chemical composition to human sebum and nourishes hair where the sebum is insufficient due either to dietary imbalances or clogging of the sebaceous glands. A nightly scalp massage will certainly nourish what hair is present and may encourage new growth. The massage, itself, will bring circulation to the scalp and may aid the restorative process.

GRAPE SEED OIL • Recently touted for their antioxidant benefits, grape seeds yield an oil which is light and nearly odorless. Grape seed oil is easily absorbed by the skin and has astringent properties which tighten and tone all types of skin.

RICE BRAN OIL • Pressed from the fibrous portion of the rice husk, rice bran oil contains plant sterols and waxes which have been shown to have an anabolic and cholesterol-reducing effect on the body. Rich in the Omega-6 fatty acids, rice bran oil lacks only alpha-linolenic acid (LNA) to complete its fatty acid profile. Note that the heaviness of this oil may cause it to penetrate the skin slowly, and its dark color may stain clothing.

WHEAT GERM OIL • Derived from the germ of the wheat grain, unrefined wheat germ oil is a nutrient-dense oil which is often rancid by the time it reaches the consumer. A bitter taste or smell indicates rancidity. The fresh oil is rich in Vitamin E and Octocosanol, two important endurance factors, as well as EFAs and other trace nutrients. A dark, 'sticky' substance, wheat germ oil often provides amazing results on diseased or troubled areas of the skin such as eczema, psoriasis, cracks, or scar tissue.

CASTOR OIL • One of the few nutritive oils derived from a bean, castor oil has been used as a traditional folk remedy for generations. Edgar Cayce popularized the use of castor oil as a detoxifying agent for the liver, gallbladder and digestive system when applied topically as a warm emollient pack. Castor oil is unique in several respects. It is the only available hydroxy vegetable oil, with 89-90% of its content Ricinoleic Acid. As a result, it has less EFAs than most vegetable oils, is more stable in terms of rancidity, and is less acidic. However, because Ricino-

Fatty Acid Content of Nutritive and Specialty Oils

Oil	Super-unsaturated Omega-3	Poly-unsaturated Omega-6	Mono-unsaturated Omega-9	Saturated
Almond		○	●	○
Apricot Kernel		◐	●	○
Borage*		●	◐	○
Canola	○	◐	●	○
Castor		○	●	
Evening Primrose*		●	○	○
Flax	●	○	○	○
Grape Seed		●	○	○
Hemp*	●	●	○	○
Jojoba			●	
Neem		◐	●	◐
Olive		○	●	○
Pumpkin	○	●	◐	○
Rice Bran		◐	●	○
Rose Hip	◐	●	○	○
Safflower		●	○	○
Sesame		●	●	○
Soybean	○	●	◐	○
Sunflower		●	◐	○
Wheat Germ	○	●	◐	○

Key:　○ = 5–19%　◐ = 20–39%　● = 40–99%

*Source of gamma-linolenic acid (GLA)

leic Acid is a strong laxative and purging agent, castor oil should not be used on a daily basis over a considerable period of time.

APRICOT KERNEL OIL • The pits of apricots yield a rich nutritive oil which is high in oleic acid and Beta Carotene. This monounsaturated oil is particularly helpful for dry, mature and sensitive skin types.

NEEM OIL • Like tea tree oil, neem oil has many remarkable topical and internal applications. Neem oil is pressed from the seeds of the neem tree which grows in low-lying tropical areas, and it has particular components which make it anti-microbial and healing. Native to India, neem has been used traditionally to heal infections of the skin and scalp, to treat tooth decay and gum diseases, to repel insects, to cure parasitic conditions in humans and animals, and as a basis for natural birth control. For more information, see Erasmus' description in *Fats That Heal, Fats That Kill*.

There are several oils which should not be used for Hygienic Oil Therapy or ingested in any form. Mineral Oil is a petroleum by-product and does not have nutritive benefits like food-source oils. Cotton Seed Oil is extracted from cotton seeds which have been sprayed with highly toxic chemicals. Cotton seeds also contain naturally-occurring toxic components which make them harmful for absorption or ingestion. Peanut Oil, while a natural food product, can be problematic due to a fungus that grows on the peanuts which, together with its carcinogenic by-products called aflatoxins, may be transferred to the oil. Other than these, virtually all oils which are pressed from healthy food products and left in an unrefined state have nutritional value.

One final point you should consider in making your selection of nutritional oils is the climate and season in which you are applying them. Because EFAs are sensitive to light as well as heat and oxygen, it is not recommended that you sunbathe for at least an hour after your oil massage unless you use a tropical oil or fat like coconut oil, cocoa butter or shea butter. Each of these is more stable than the oils previously mentioned and will not break down or rancidify in the heat and sunlight.

Apart from sunbathing, try to select an oil which suits your local climate and season. Oils like flax, safflower, canola, and sunflower, which contain a higher percent of unsaturated fatty acids, are suited to climates and seasons which are cooler and have less sunlight. To avoid oxidation, it is best to use them on areas of the skin that will be covered by clothing. Oils like olive, almond and sesame, however, which contain more of the stable monounsaturates, are suited to climates and seasons which are warmer and sunnier. They are also more appropriate to use on areas of unprotected skin. Use your intelligence and intuition to select an oil or blend of oils which agrees with you and your environment.

> *"Anoint one's interior with honey*
> *and one's exterior with oil"*
>
> —Democritus, when asked how to
> live long and maintain good health.

CHAPTER 5

Your Daily Oil Massage

"For most Romans, a visit to the baths was the highlight of their day. . . . Afterward (baths and steam) an attendant oiled his (the bather's) body and scraped it with a strigil to remove sweat and dirt . . . the citizen departed, refreshed in body and spirit."

—From *Greece and Rome: Builders of our World*

We now come to the most important and personal part of this book: your daily oil massage. It is important because this is what you need to do to realize any benefits—what you read will not add any EFAs to your body! It is personal because there is really no 'right' or 'wrong' way to do it. It is best, therefore, to do it in a way that is comfortable for you and to try to make it a part of your daily hygienic practice, like brushing your teeth or combing your hair. As with these healthy habits, the benefit is in the doing. You will look better and feel better for allowing the ten minutes each day it takes to perform. What happens if you only have five minutes? Abbreviate the massage. You will still gain important health benefits.

Instead of describing an elaborate routine, I will simply tell you what I do each day and offer some variations for you to consider. The rest is up to you to follow or to improvise as you wish.

My 'routine' consists of two parts: a morning 'after-shower' oil massage of my body, arms, legs, hands and feet and a 'before-bed' oil massage of my scalp, face and neck. I do both after I wash with a high-quality castile soap which removes the sweat, dirt and grime that have accumulated during the day or night. I often use organic, cold-pressed olive oil, although I have come to prefer sesame or flax oil in the cooler seasons. I have also enjoyed experimenting with some of the other nutritive oils, including a richly-scented blend which offers a full spectrum of EFAs.

In the morning, after I walk a mile or two, I usually eat a piece (or two) of fresh fruit or drink a glass of fresh juice. Next, I enjoy a warm shower and wash myself thoroughly. Afterwards, I dry myself with a towel, being careful to leave a little moisture on my skin. (Warmth and a little moisture help the oil to spread and to be absorbed by the skin.)

Next, I pour a bit of the warmed oil[1] into the palms of one or both of my hands and begin rubbing it onto my skin. I usually begin with my feet and work my way up. The order is relatively unimportant, however, compared to covering the entire body (except the head) with a light film of oil.

On my limbs, I use longer and straighter strokes while, on my body, I use more rounded strokes. I generally follow the therapeutic guideline of massaging toward the center of the body, the heart. I also follow a crossover pattern on the front and top parts of my body according to the theory of polarity[2] as described below. This process is also an interesting experience in getting to know my own body. Why not accept it as it is even as I make choices for positive health? Once I have finished

---

[1]A simple way to warm the oil you are going to use is to put a few tablespoons of oil into a cup immediately prior to showering or bathing. Using warm to mildly hot tap water, fill a small pan, half-full, and place the cup of oil into the pan of water. As you shower, the oil will warm, treating you to a more relaxing massage afterward.

[2]The theory of polarity is a part of what is sometimes called "energy medicine." It holds that life is a dynamic state of flux between opposite poles of energy. According to this theory, different sides of the body represent different poles or charges. Touching the body can establish either a subtle circuit or short-circuit, depending on the relationship of the parts touched. The right hand is considered to be paired with the left (front) side of the body, and the left hand is considered to be paired with the right (front) side. According to Dr. Robert C. Fulford in his book, *Dr. Fulford's Touch of Life* (Pocket Books, 1996), "this applies only to the sensory portion of the human body, or the front side, and not the body's motor section, or the back." I have found this crossover pattern, as suggested by Dr. Fulford, to be extremely beneficial in Hygienic Oil Therapy.

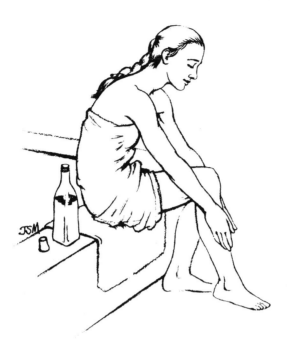

Hygienic Oil Therapy: Your Daily Self-Massage

with the massage, I give the oil a minute or two to 'soak in' and then I get dressed.

You may have a problem or two with this routine and wish to vary it accordingly. If excess oil is left on the skin, it may stain or scent your clothing. Whites and undergarments are particularly liable to be stained. If this is a problem for you, I would suggest that you perform the oil massage before your shower as Deepak Chopra suggests. This accomplishes less, however, since the soap that you wash with will emulsify most of the oil and thus remove it. Also, in all of the ancient traditions, bathing preceded anointment. As an alternative, you might consider using a lighter color of oil. Or you might relax a few minutes longer until the oil soaks thoroughly into your skin.

You may find that some of the oil gets spilled onto the floor or into the sink. Keeping an old towel handy makes cleaning up easy. Be sure to wipe off any oil that spills into your sink, as it can often clog the drain.

Anoint Yourself With Oil For Radiant Health

My nightly routine is intended to cover my head and face which were omitted from the morning routine. The reason I chose to omit them was because I do not look particularly attractive (or so I think!) with oil in my hair or on my face. Also, I seem to sleep more soundly when I allow the oil to soak into my scalp at night. The downside, of course, is my pillow case which may be stained by the oil. As a result, I use an old sheepskin covering on the outside of my pillow.

In any case, my nightly routine follows the same wash-and-massage pattern as my morning routine. I wash my face, hands, and neck with a natural olive or castille soap, and then I apply the oil. On my face, I follow the contours and lines, spreading the oil and massaging lightly.

Next, I massage the oil into my scalp, using just enough so that my hair and scalp are covered with a light film. If too much oil is used, it can easily be toweled off. This nightly routine is also a journey of discovery as I feel the contours of my face and look at myself in the mirror. Who do I see today?

Once again, this routine is only my personal habit. Whatever habit or choices meet your needs are entirely up to you. The important thing is to do what works best. If you only do the oil massage in the winter, you will still benefit in the most appropriate season. If you are a night person, try setting up a nightly routine. Whatever works.

"For the Lord Your God is bringing you into a good land . . . a land of olive oil and honey."

—Deut. 8:7, 8

CHAPTER 6

Aromatherapy and Oils

*"The odors of ointments are more
durable than those of flowers."*

—Sir Francis Bacon, *Of Praise.*

There are many fine books available which can give you detailed information on the science and art of using essential oils. In a brief chapter, I can only outline some of the guiding principals on the subject and list a few of the beneficial properties of the most popular oils.

The tradition of perfuming is as ancient as the tradition of pressing oils. The two have often been used together to enhance their individual therapeutic and aesthetic benefits. The word 'perfume' comes to us from the Latin and literally means, 'through the smoke,' since it was originally applied to incense as well as to fragrant oils.

There is a religious tradition involving the use of fragrance which runs parallel to the tradition of anointment with oil. Fragrant incenses and perfumes have been employed in the religious practices of the Egyptian, Greek, Hindu, Japanese, Haitian, Buddhist, Hebrew and Christian traditions, as well as many others. Mohammed considered perfume to be one of the supreme delights, and his vision of paradise was rich with exotic scents. In addition, perfumes and fumigants were used to help cure the sick and cast out 'evil spirits' from diseased individuals. Not surprisingly, perfumes of various composition have been used in the hygienic and aesthetic toilet rituals of the majority of civilized cultures. Perhaps perfume's most fabled usage has been as an aphrodisiac and emblem of love in furthering the attraction of the sexes.

Essential oils were originally derived from flowers and plants which were rubbed directly onto the skin. Since the invention of the steam distillation process, this has been the primary method of extracting essential oils. Newer methods, such as cold-pressing, enfleurage, solvent-extraction, turbo-distillation, hydrodiffusion and carbon dioxide extraction are also currently in use. Of these, only solvent-extracted essences should be ruled out from among the products you choose. As I stated earlier, the toxic chemicals used in this extractive process makes these oils unsuitable for topical or internal use. It should also be noted that many essences are now synthesized. Since these synthetics cannot duplicate the complex and synergistic balances of the volatile oils nature included in each plant, they are hygienically inferior to natural essences and are usually more harmful than healthy.

Beyond these guidelines, the quality of essential oils are entirely dependent on the skill and care that was applied to their creation. Please be sensitive to this fact, and buy only the highest quality essences from manufacturers who have earned your trust. And trust your own instincts! If you react negatively to an essential oil, do not use it. It probably has little or no therapeutic value.

The therapeutic benefits of Aromatherapy can be great where the essential oils used are natural and of the highest quality. These oils have distinct, "clean" aromas, and the recognition of their source is immediate and pleasant, like a fond childhood memory. Acting directly upon the olfactory nerves of the brain, they can either be powerful stimulants or relaxants, and their usage can greatly enhance the therapeutic benefits of Hygienic Oil Therapy. To use them, simply place a few drops of the essential oil in your nutritive oil prior to your daily oil massage.

Here are some popular oils and a few of their traditionally-recognized benefits:

ANISE • This oil is derived from anise seeds and has a pleasant, licorice-like aroma. It is mildly-stimulating and useful to promote perspiration.

BASIL • The oil of basil leaves is sweet-smelling and mildly spicy. Considered the "King of plants" by the Greeks, basil was an important ingredient in the anointing oil of Kings. Basil is useful for colds, respiratory problems, digestive problems, arthritis and fatigue. Generally speaking, basil strengthens the nerves.

BERGAMOT • Taken from the bergamot tree, this oil is both sweet and citrus-like in its aroma. Its antiseptic properties make it useful in healing urinary tract infections, cold sores and shingles. It is considered "refreshing and uplifting."

CAMPHOR • This oil is very strong in scent and activity. Derived from the stems of the leaves of camphor trees, camphor oil is used to treat colds and flus, injuries, shock, trauma and anxiety. It is a strong stimulant with antiseptic and analgesic properties.

CEDARWOOD • Cedarwood oil is distilled from the wood of cedar trees. Its astringent properties give it value in treating skin eruptions. It is also a diuretic, expectorant and mild sedative.

CHAMOMILE • Chamomile flowers are used to distill this light and pleasant-smelling oil. Its cooling properties are useful in reducing fever and every sort of inflammation. It calms the nerves, helps to reduce stress, and aids relaxation.

CINNAMON • The warming properties of cinnamon oil assist circulation. It is also both astringent and relaxing.

CITRONELLA • Derived from citronella grass, the lemony-scent of this oil is useful in the summertime to keep the insects away.

CLARY SAGE • Clary sage oil is obtained from a variety of sage leaves and the flowering tops of the plant. It has a sweet, fresh, clean and warm scent with an undertone of balsam.

CLOVE • Clove is a warming oil with mild analgesic properties. Distilled from clove buds, this aromatic oil was used to relieve toothaches long before oral analgesics were invented.

EUCALYPTUS • Eucalyptus is renowned for its stimulating properties in relieving respiratory problems, colds and flus, fevers and local congestion due to injury. The oil of Eucalyptus leaves is emotionally refreshing and is known to possess anti-microbial activity and relieve pain.

GINGER • Pungent and warming, ginger oil comes from the roots of ginger plants. A traditional remedy for nausea, ginger's warming prop-

Anoint Yourself With Oil For Radiant Health

erties bring a ruddiness to the skin. As a digestive oil, its uses are more internal than external.

JASMINE • The light scent of Jasmine flowers makes this oil an excellent choice for relaxation as well as lifting the spirits. A hormone balancer, jasmine is useful for both women's and men's problems.

JUNIPER • Derived from juniper berries, this oil was used by the Egyptians to anoint themselves. Juniper helps fight urinary tract infections, eases menstrual disorders, relieves arthritis and digestive disorders and helps to minimize stress.

LAVENDER • Lavender blossoms yield a sweet-smelling floral oil which is regarded as calming and relaxing yet strengthening to the nerves. Its mildness assists many disorders, including skin problems, sore throats, headaches and child- hood illnesses.

LEMON • The astringent properties of lemon peel make this an excellent oil for fighting infection, aiding digestion, cooling fever, soothing and toning the skin and refreshing and uplifting the spirit.

LIME • The peels of limes offers many of the same benefits as lemon with a distinctly refreshing, clean aroma.

MYRRH • The sweet, warm, spicy scent of myrrh is unique among essential oils. Distilled from the resins of the bark of the myrrh bush, this oil has a noted history as part of the biblical anointing oil. Myrrh is useful in boosting immunity and speeding recovery from illness. It is used for gum disorders and other internal and topical infections. Myrrh oil is considered to be exceptional for maintaining healthy skin and fortifying the nerves.

ORANGE • From whole oranges or their peels, orange oil is either pressed or distilled. The citrus aroma of oranges is both normalizing and stimulating and is useful in treating infections, boosting immunity and restoring balance to dry or oily skin.

PATCHOULI • The earthy, exotic, spicy scent of patchouli is obtained from the dried and fermented leaves of the Patchouli plant. Patchouli is considered a relaxant, tonic and aphrodisiac. It is reported to aid in weight loss and skin cell regeneration. India and Southeast Asia provide the origins of this oil.

PENNYROYAL • This oil is derived from European pennyroyal flowers. Its scent can be used to fight colds or as a fragrance. As a digestive agent, it expels gas and, externally, it brings circulation to the skin.

PEPPERMINT • This oil is cool, refreshing and uplifting. Distilled from peppermint leaves, it has a stimulating effect wherever it is used. It also has antiseptic properties. Peppermint oil strengthens the central nervous system and relaxes the smooth muscles of the digestive tract.

PINE • 'The strong, fresh, balsamic' scent of pine needles characterize an oil that is useful in treating any type of respiratory infection, warming a chill or cooling a fever, and easing muscle or joint pains. Its vitalizing effect is systemic and may cause an increase in blood pressure.

ROSE • The rose has been the subject of art, literature, poetry, myth and song throughout history. As an emblem of love, a rose's scent is considered to soothe all the emotions. Rose oil has been used to treat a wide variety of conditions, including cold sores, digestive disorders, female problems, sexual difficulties and outbreaks of the skin.

ROSEMARY • Distilled from the leaves of the blossoming rosemary plant, rosemary oil has a "pungent pine-like aroma with a woody, camphorous note." Herbalists have recommended rosemary to stimulate the activity of the stomach, the liver, the gallbladder and to improve circulation.

SANDALWOOD • This pale or golden-colored oil is distilled from the heartwood of the sandalwood tree. The sandalwood is an evergreen which grows in Coastal areas of India. Its scent is rich, warm, and sweet with exotic overtones. Sandalwood oil has been traditionally used in the spiritual practices of India for thousands of years and is considered to awaken the life force of its users. Medicinally, it has been helpful in cases of infection, particularly of the urinary tract, and also congestive problems. Sandalwood oil has been prized as an aphrodisiac and is considered to have calming properties.

SASSAFRAS • Sassafras has a rich heritage of usage within the American herbal tradition as a spring cleaning tonic, and the oil of the sassafras bark shares many of the same cleansing and warming properties. A spicy scent, not unlike root beer, adds to the warm, woody bouquet of this oil.

SPEARMINT • Cool, light and stimulating, the aroma of spearmint oil is useful for lifting the spirits and refreshing the body. Spearmint oil shares many of the therapeutic benefits of peppermint and wintergreen.

TANGERINE • This oil is cold pressed, rather than distilled, from the peels of tangerines. It has a light, sweet, tangy scent which is both uplifting and fortifying.

TEA TREE • Tea tree oil is a medicinal oil which is distilled from the leaves of a single species of the tea tree family. These trees grow primarily in southeastern Australia. The oil's scent is strong, pungent and spicy and resembles that of its botanical cousin, the eucalyptus. Tea tree oil has many important therapeutic applications owing to its potent antiseptic properties. It is useful in treating all infectious conditions, both internal and external. It has been used to heal cuts, wounds and burns by native Aborigines for centuries. It has also proven itself to be invaluable in treating most respiratory conditions, since it acts as an expectorant as well as a antimicrobial agent. Tea tree oil is known to heal many skin conditions, including acne and fungal infections of the nails. Its scent is stimulating but it can also center the emotions in times of stress or trauma.

THYME OIL • Thyme leaves have traditionally been associated with courage. Like courage, the oil of thyme has many applications. Its warm and spicy scent fights infections, improves immunity, increases circulation, and strengthens the nerves.

WINTERGREEN OIL • One of the coolest of the oils, wintergreen, like peppermint and spearmint, is derived from the leaves of the plant and shares many of their stimulating, fever-reducing properties.

YLANG-YLANG OIL • This relaxing, sweet oil is distilled from the exotic flowers of the Ylang-Ylang Tree. For hundreds of years, people of tropical cultures have scented coconut oil with Ylang-Ylang to enhance the beauty of their skin and hair. Ylang-Ylang oil is soothing, calming and sensual.

Aryuvedic Combinations

In Chapter 2, we introduced the Aryuvedic tradition of abhyanga or the daily oil massage. Aryuveda also uses essential oils and herbs to treat specific imbalances in the system according to the principle of Doshas or body types. The three primary types are Vata, Pitta and Kapha, as we have already discussed. According to Deepak Chopra's interpretation of the tradition, the thin, quick, cold and dry Vata types are best balanced by scents which are "warm, sweet and sour." Examples are: basil, rose geranium, clove, anise, fennel, licorice and thyme. He recommends "sweet, cool aromas" for the hot, sharp, moist, and sour Pitta dosha. These include rose, mint, sandalwood, cinnamon and jasmine. Finally, the heavy, sweet, steady, soft and slow Kapha type are best balanced by scents which are "warm, but with spicier overtones." He recommends "juniper, eucalyptus, camphor, clove and marjoram." For a detailed discussion of Doshas, Sub-Doshas, Abhyanga and Aromatherapy, please refer to Dr. Chopra's book, *Perfect Health.*

Of course, it is also possible to select and add your own choice of essential oils to your daily oil massage. If you are sensitive, you may wish to leave your oil massage free of aroma except for the delicate scents of the oils themselves. Again, trust your instincts to make the choices you require for health.

> *"Venus at the approach of twilight returned from the banquet of the gods, breathing odors and crowned with roses."*
>
> —from *Bullfinch's Mythology,*
> Cupid and Psyche

CHAPTER 7

Fasting and Oil Therapy

*"When you fast, anoint your head
and wash your face"*

—Mt. 6:16

Fasting for ritual purification and spiritual enlightenment is a practice which is as ancient and universal as anointment with oil and perfumery with flowers and herbs. The ability to function without eating for considerable periods of time was essential for survival in hunter-gatherer cultures, and the caloric value of fats and oils were appreciated in this context. The religious practice of self-denial through fasting, in all likelihood, was an unconscious reminder of those ancient times when the spirits of animals or the vegetative earth were invoked to provide sustenance for the tribe. At the same time, primitive people may have observed the mental clarity their fasts brought them and would also have been more in touch with the animal instinct to turn away from food during times of illness and stress. Together, these forces shaped the practice of fasting within more "civilized" cultures where it became ritualized and symbolic as well as practical and hygienic.

The practice of fasting has been employed in nearly every religion known to man. In ancient times, the cults of Isis and Osiris practiced ritual fasting as well as those discussed in the Eleusinian Mysteries. The American Plains Indians fasted in order to purify themselves and prepare for their dance before the Great Spirit. In the Hebrew tradition, fasting was associated with atonement and communion with Yaweh, their God. The forty day fast of Jesus has been an example to Christians of a way to dedicate, purify and prepare for communion with their Heavenly Father. The Eastern religions of Hinduism, Buddhism and Islam also have rich traditions of fasting which were typified by the purifying fasts of the Buddha and Mohammed. Within the Hindu tradition, Mahatma Gandhi adapted the practice of fasting to protest political injustice as well as to inform his own conscience and to increase his spiritual awareness.

One of the early instances where fasting and anointment are coupled is given in II Samuel 12:16-23. This passage recounts King David's fast during the illness of his son by Bathsheba. His fast is broken after seven days when his child dies. David's acceptance of this death is described as follows: "So David arose from the ground, washed and anointed himself and changed his clothes; and he went into the house of the Lord and worshipped."

In recent times, fasting has been employed for purposes of health and hygiene, apart from religious ritual or tradition. Its many adherents have taught that fasting is a way to cleanse the system of accumulated toxins and their associated physical and emotional effects. In particular, fasting allows the bowels to be cleansed and healed, offers a rest to the overworked liver and kidneys in their detoxifying roles, and stimulates the breakdown of fat tissue and the release of fat-bound toxins within the system. Two excellent books on this subject are *Rational Fasting* by Professor Arnold Ehret and *Fasting Can Save Your Life* by Herbert M. Shelton. Both men recommend supervision of fasts by qualified professionals in order to avoid unpleasant side effects and to minimize traumatic healing crises.

I first began to perform oil massages on myself when I was on a seven day water and juice fast. Because the levels of contaminants and toxins in my system were at significant levels, this was undoubtedly too strenuous an effort for only my second fast. Nevertheless, because I was quite ill and unable to keep food down, I pressed on.

During this time, I was miserable. My stomach cramped and ached, I had difficulty sleeping, and I nearly passed out each time I got out of bed. By the end of the fast, I had to concentrate almost entirely on vegetable juices, or I think I might have ended up in the hospital.

The other saving grace for me was my daily oil massage. I was quite thin and needed some calories in my system. The water and juices I drank did little to keep the cold of the Midwestern winter out of my bones. Yet the oil massage really helped. After a warm shower and massage, I felt stronger, more calm and relaxed, and better prepared to work rather than simply rest. These benefits occurred even while I was giving my digestive system a chance to heal and ridding myself of a large portion of forty years of accumulated wastes and toxins.

Looking back, I would not attempt a fast beyond three days without qualified supervision. Prof. Ehret recommends three days as a reasonable period to begin with in order to determine the level of a person's toxicity. The more debilitated a person feels during these three days, he states, the more serious is their condition. He also observes that the more serious conditions require both proper supervision and a gradual rather than a heroic detoxification.

What science is beginning to understand is that the skin is an organ of metabolism and not just a passive barrier or an organ of elimination. It is capable of providing a measure of nourishment to the system, and its own nourishment provides rest for the system as a whole. Hygienic Oil Therapy is thus a vital component in any fasting or detoxification program. Nourishment comes through the gradual metabolic processes of the skin while the digestive organs rest. And the healthy EFAs provided by nutritional oils are perhaps the most important nutrients to obtain during a fast. The healing crisis is softened and eased by the important benefits of these nutrients. Perhaps this is why anointment with oil is traditionally and symbolically linked to fasting and a renewal of the spirit. Both are important and therapeutic.

> *"If the brain and the belly are burn-*
> *ing clean with fasting, every moment*
> *a new song comes out of the fire"*
>
> —Rumi, from "Fasting"

CHAPTER 8

Questions and Answers

"Thou anointest my head with oil"

—Ps. 23:5

Q **If my skin itches or breaks out when I apply the oil, what should I do?**

A Itching indicates an irritant, either in the skin or in the oil. Try switching to an organic, unrefined oil, preferably in a glass container. If the itching persists, the problem is most likely in the skin. In this case, the oil therapy should gradually reduce the itching. A medically-supervised fast may also be helpful.

Q **Will I gain weight if I perform the oil massage each day?**

A Perhaps a little, particularly if you are thin to begin with. People in the normal range should have no problem since the oil represents a small fraction of their daily caloric intake. Moreover, unrefined oil contains healthy fat which will help to 'stoke the furnace' of your cellular metabolism. Consequently, you may actually lose weight in the long term. Obese individuals often have more serious metabolic problems which should be addressed by a holistic health care professional. The oil therapy can be a valuable adjunct to a medically-supervised fast for these individuals and can help to reduce their cravings for sweets, simple starches and unhealthy fats. A change in diet and lifestyle is required, of which the oil therapy can be a valuable part.

Q **What should I do if I have a skin condition such as acne, eczema or psoriasis?**

A These conditions require medical supervision by a qualified holistic health care practitioner. Once again, a supervised fast may be helpful. In the long-term, the oil therapy can be tremendously beneficial to nearly all conditions of the skin. You may wish to avoid putting the oil directly onto any lesions if the pain it causes is excessive. Oils such as evening primrose, flax, borage, black current, neem, and olive have nutritive properties which can be quite beneficial to these conditions. Often, they can be applied directly onto the lesions.

Q **What kind of oil should I use?**

A   The variety of oil is your choice — See Chapter 4. However, olive or sesame are two traditional choices with excellent healing properties. I also highly recommend unrefined flax, hemp and sunflower oils. Whatever variety of oil you choose, try to use an organic, unrefined oil, Its nutritional profile will be superior to a refined product and you will not need to worry about pesticide or solvent residues.

Q **How soon will I start to see benefits?**

A   Hygienic Oil Therapy is a healthy habit, and its benefits will be gradually revealed as the body rids itself of unwanted toxins, and the healthy fats begin to offset the unhealthy ones. A dietary reform is an important adjunct — away from processed sugars, starches, fats and chemicals and toward natural whole foods. This being said, most people feel better after they perform their first oil massage — and every time subsequently.

Q **I am an active athlete. Will the oil therapy affect my performance in any way?**

A   According to Udo Erasmus, Ph.D., healthy fats (unsaturated) will enhance your performance while unhealthy fats (saturated or hydrogenated) will hinder it. He states, "the fats that heal are required for healthy oxidation, energy production, regulation of cell function and healing of tissue injuries, sprains and bruises. The fats that kill interfere with health and slow down athletic performances." Based on the chain length of the fatty acids in Olive Oil and Coconut Oil, these are excellent choices for providing sustained energy during an athletic event. Coconut Oil has cooling properties which make it well suited for warmer weather, and it provides the energy-rich MCT's (Medium Chain Triglycerides) for sustained endurance. Try the oil therapy in training and I'm sure you will insist upon a pre-event oil massage.

Q   **I have developed brown "spots" on my skin after starting the Hygienic Oil Therapy. What are they and how do I get rid of them?**

A   These spots or blotches are stains of the skin from the plant pigments of some of the darker, richer unrefined oils. They are completely harmless and will wear off in a few days or a week. You can speed the process of removing them by brushing your skin with a loofa while you are showering or bathing. Try switching to a lighter-colored oil.

Q   **Is there anything else I can do to enhance the benefits of Hygienic Oil Therapy?**

A   Yes. It is helpful to ensure that your intake of antioxidants is sufficient to balance the increased intake of nutritional oils. Because these oils help to "stoke the furnace" of your cells through the process of oxidation, the antioxidants are needed to insure that the "fire" does not get out of control and cause damage to your cells. Some of these antioxidants are: the vitamins A, C and E, the minerals Zinc and Selenium, the enzyme Superoxide Dismutase (SOD), and the amino acids L-Cysteine and L-Glutathione. Pine Bark Extract (Pycnogenol) and Grape See Extract also contain naturally-occurring flavonoid compounds, known as proanthocyanidins, which are powerful antioxidants.

One of the advantages of using unrefined nutritional oil is that some of these antioxidants are preserved, through careful processing, in the finished product and are available to nourish your skin and body.

In addition, it is beneficial to insure that you consume adequate quantities of the nutrients necessary to convert EFAs to prostaglandins: Vitamin C, B_3 and B_6 as well as Zinc and Magnesium.

> *"Everything is soothed by oil . . .*
> *it soothes every rough part."*
>
> —Pliny, The Elder

"And once the surf
had scoured the thick caked sweat from their limbs
and the two fighters cooled, their hearts revived
and into the polished tubs they climbed and bathed.
And rinsing off, their skin sleek with an olive oil rub,
they sat down to their meal."

—Homer's *The Illiad,* Book X, 663-668

"Meanwhile, the lovely Polykaste, youngest daughter
of Nestor, the son of Neleus, washed Telemachos
And when she had washed him and anointed him
*   richly with oil,*
she put a lovely mantle on him and a tunic.
And he left the bathtub in body like the immortals.

—Homer's *The Odyssey,* Book III, 464-468

Sources of Oil

Nutritional Oil Products

Now Foods
550 Mitchell Rd.
Glendale Heights, IL 60139
(630) 545-9098

Arrowhead Mills, Inc.
110 South Lawton St.
Hereford, TX 79045
364-0730

Spectrum Naturals
133 Copeland Street
Petaluma, CA 94952
278-8900

Flora, Inc.
805 E. Badger Road
Lyndon., WA 98264
(360) 354-2110

Barleans Organic Oils
4936 Lake Torrell Road
Ferndale, WA 98248
(800) 445-3529

The Ohio Hempery, Inc.
P.O. Box 18
Guysville, OH 45731
(800) BUY-HEMP

Omega Nutrition
6505 Ardvich Road
Bellingham, WA 98226
(604) 253-4677

Health From The Sun
962 Rte. 11
Sunapee, NY 03782
(603) 763-4745

Aromatherapy Products

Now Foods
550 Mitchell Rd.
Glendale Heights, IL 60139
(630) 545-9098

Aura Cacia
101 Paymaster Road
Weaverville, CA 96093
(800) 437-3301

The Essential Oil Company
P.O. Box 206
Lake Oswego, OR 97034
697-5992

Amrita Aromatherapy, Inc.
800 N. 12th Street
Fairfield, IA 52556
(515) 472-9136

Aroma Vera
5901 Rodeo Road
Los Angeles, CA 90016-4312
280-0407

Consumer Direct

The Fruitful Yield Mail Order (800) 469-5552

APPENDIX II

Bibliography

Balch, James F., MD, and Phyllis A., C.N.C. *Prescription for Nutritional Healing.* Avery Publishing Group, Inc. Garden Park City, NY, 1990.

Brandon, S.G.F. "Oil." *Man, Myth and Magic.* Ed. By Richard Cavendish. Marshall Cavendish Corp.: North Bellmore, New York, 1995, Vol. 14, pp. 1913, 1914.

Brown, Royden. *Bee Hive Product Bible.* Avery Publishing Group, Inc.: Garden City Park, NY, 1993.

'Cupid and Psyche'. *Bullfinch's Mythology.* Harper and Row Publishers, Inc.: New York, NY, 1970.

Chopra, Deepak, MD. *Perfect Health.* Harmony Books: NY, 1990.

Ehret, Arnold. Mucusless Diet Healing System. Ehret Literature Publishing, Co., Inc.: Yonkers, NY, 1994.

Erasmus, Udo. *Fats that Heal, Fats that Kill.* Alive Books: Burnaby, British Columbia. 1993.

Farah, Adelaide P. "Beautiful Barrier." Health, May 1986. Vol. 18, pp. 64-68.

Gorse, Leslie. "Patchwork Medicine." Science, Oct. 1985. V. 6, pp. 79, 80

Greece and Rome: Builders of Our World. National Geographic Society: Washington, DC, 1968.

Holy Bible. New King James Version. Thomas Nelson Publishers: Nashville, TN, 1982.

Homer. *The Illiad.* Transl. By Robert Fagles. Viking-Penguin: NY, 1990.

Homer. *The Odyssey.* Trans. By Albert Cook. W.W. Norton & Company, Inc. New York, NY 1974.

"Integumentary System." *Gale Encyclopedia of Science.* Ed. by Bridget Travis. Gale Research: Detroit, MI, 1966. Vol. 5, pp. 1942-1944.

Macnamara, Ellen. *The Everyday Life of the Etruscan*. Dorset Press: New York, 1973.

Maple, Eric. "Perfume." *Man, Myth and Magic*. Ed. by Richard Cavendish. Marshall Cavendish Corp: North Bellmore, NY. 1995, Vol. 15, p.p. 2008-2011.

Raloff, Janet. "Hairy Portals for Toxic Chemicals." *Science News*, June 25, 1988. N. 26, p. 407.

Rousseau, Jean Jaques. *Emil or Education*. Translation and notes by Allan Bloom. New York: Basic Books, 1979.

Sappho, translated by Mary Barnard. Shambhala Publications, Inc.: Boston, 1994.

The Columbia Dictionary of Quotations. Ed. by Robert Andrews. Columbia University Press: New York, 1993.

The Essential Rumi. translated by Coleman Barks. HarperSan Francisco, Harper-Collins: NY, 1995.

Webster's New Twentieth Century Dictionary, Second Edition. Ed. by Jean L. McKechnie. World Publishing Company: Cleveland and New York, 1966.

Wilson, Roberta. *Aromatherapy for Vibrant Health and Beauty*. Avery Publishing Group: Garden City Park, NY, 1995.

Word Mysteries and Histories. American Heritage Dictionaries. Houghton-Mifflin Company. Boston. 1986. P. 168.

World Book Rush-Presbyterian-St. Luke's Medical Center Medical Encyclopedia, 7th Ed. WorldBook, Inc., 1995.

Anoint Yourself With Oil For Radiant Health